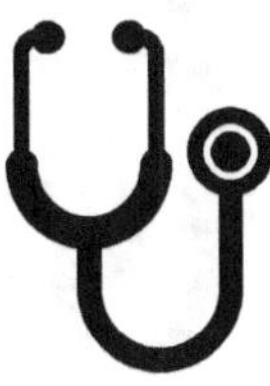

I0788082

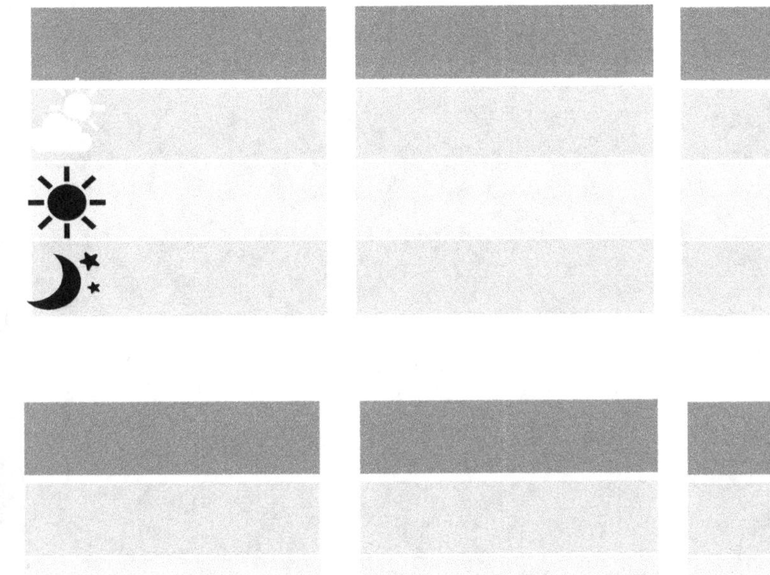

MEDICAL NOTES

MEDICAL NOTES

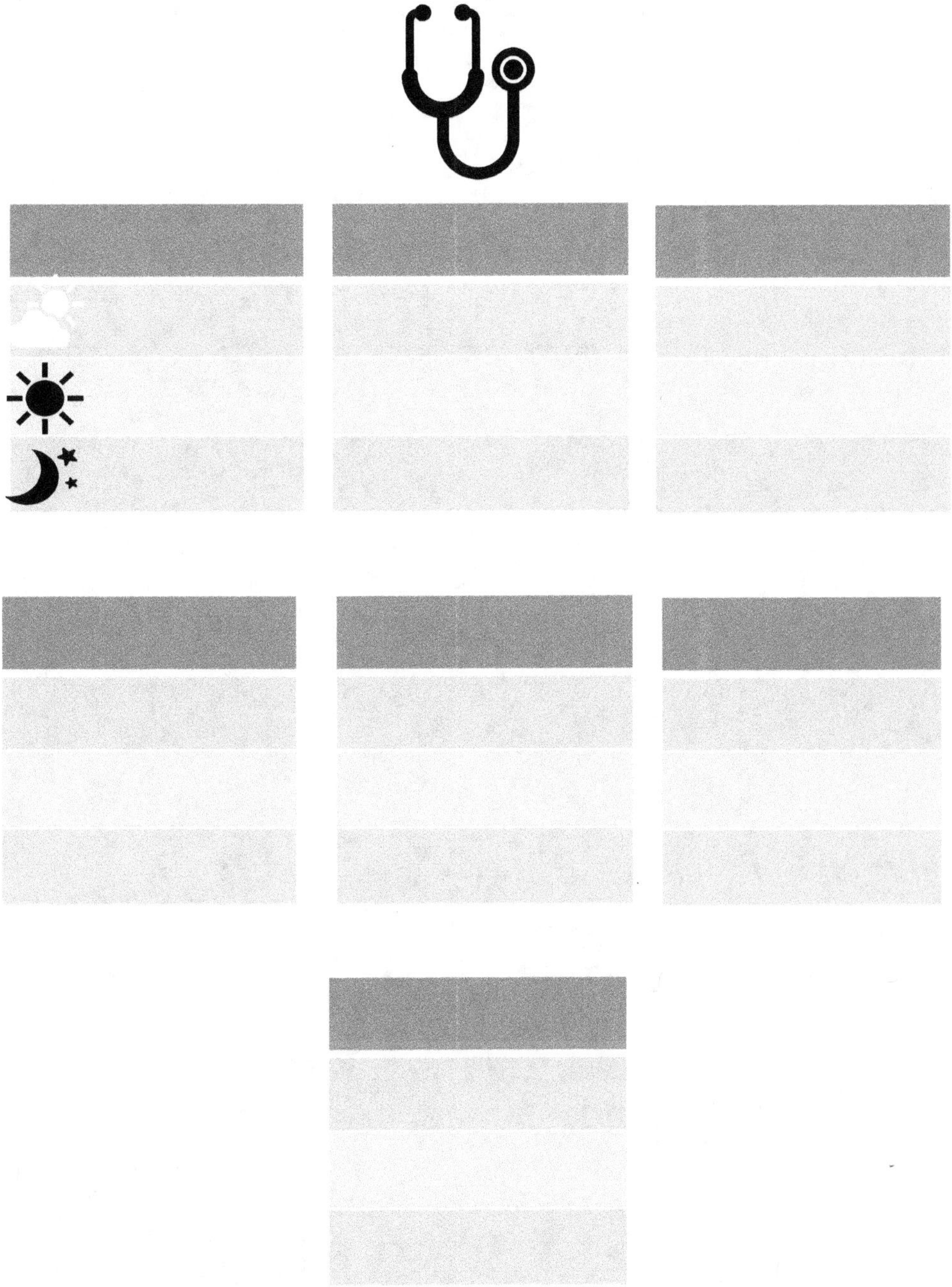

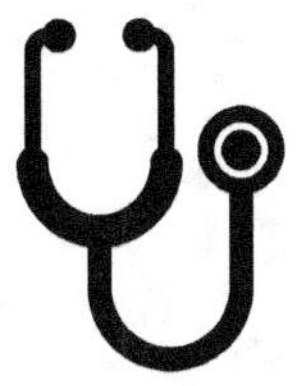

MEDICAL NOTES

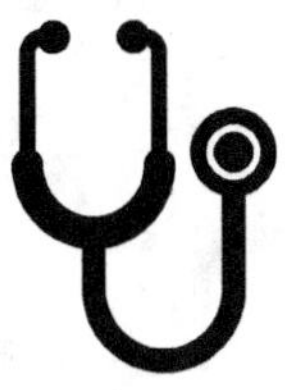

MEDICAL NOTES

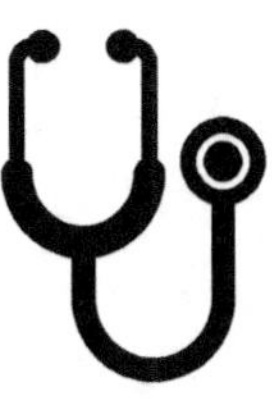

MEDICAL NOTES

MEDICAL NOTES

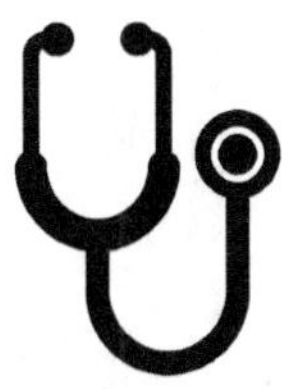

MEDICAL NOTES

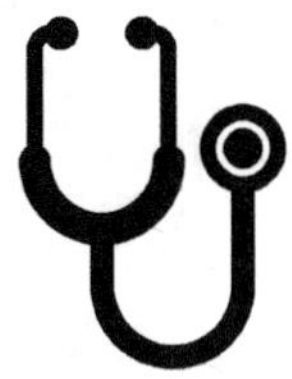

MEDICAL NOTES

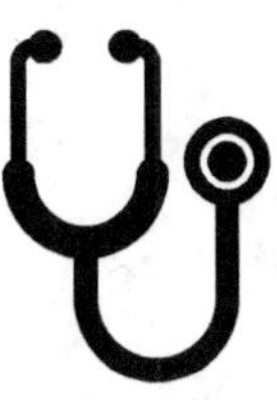

MEDICAL NOTES

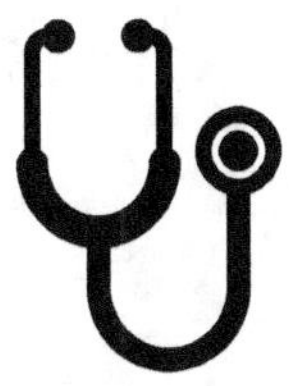

MEDICAL NOTES

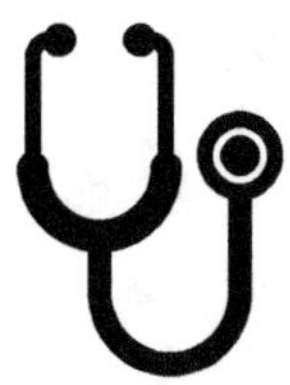

MEDICAL NOTES

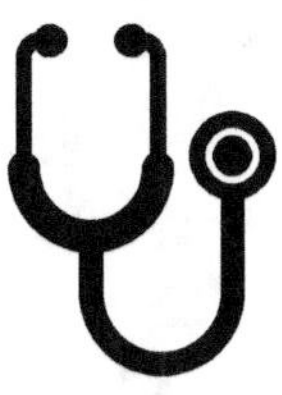

MEDICAL NOTES

MEDICAL NOTES

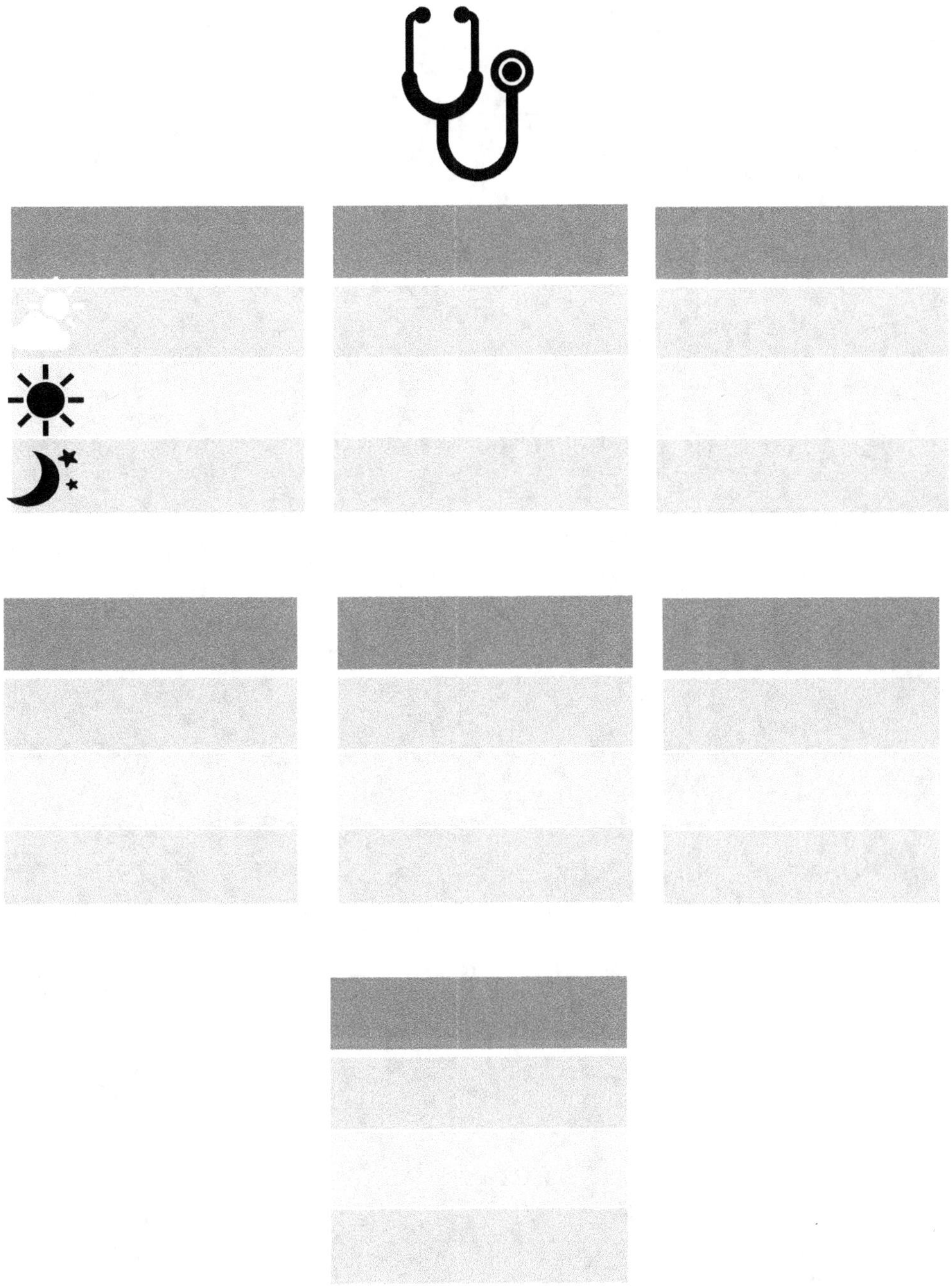

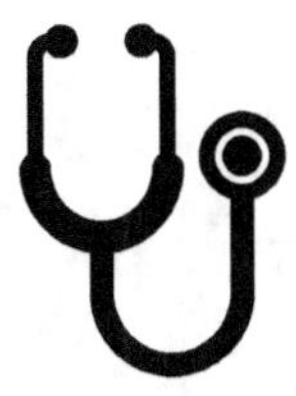

MEDICAL NOTES

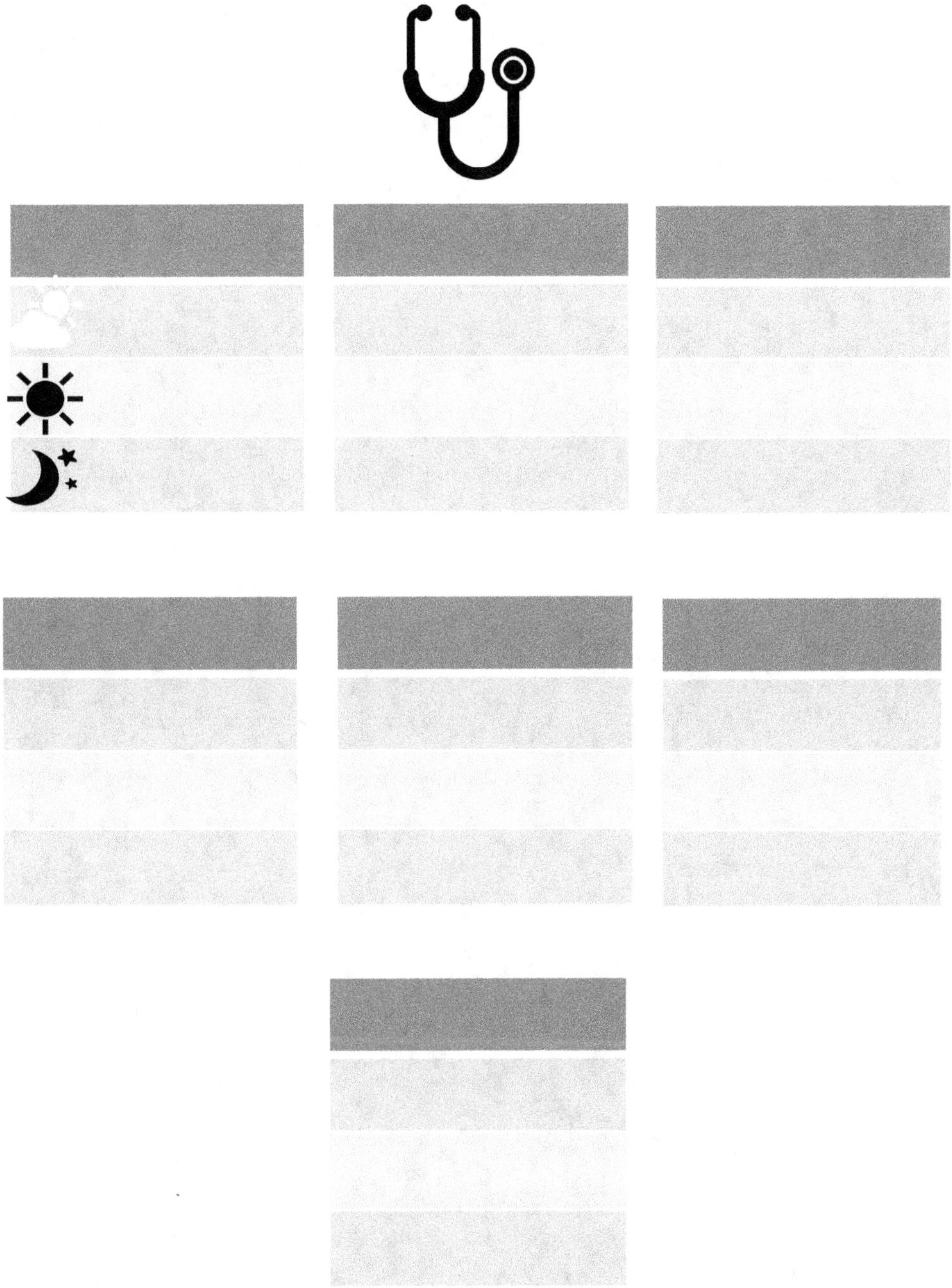

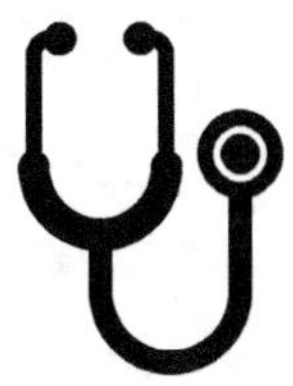

MEDICAL NOTES

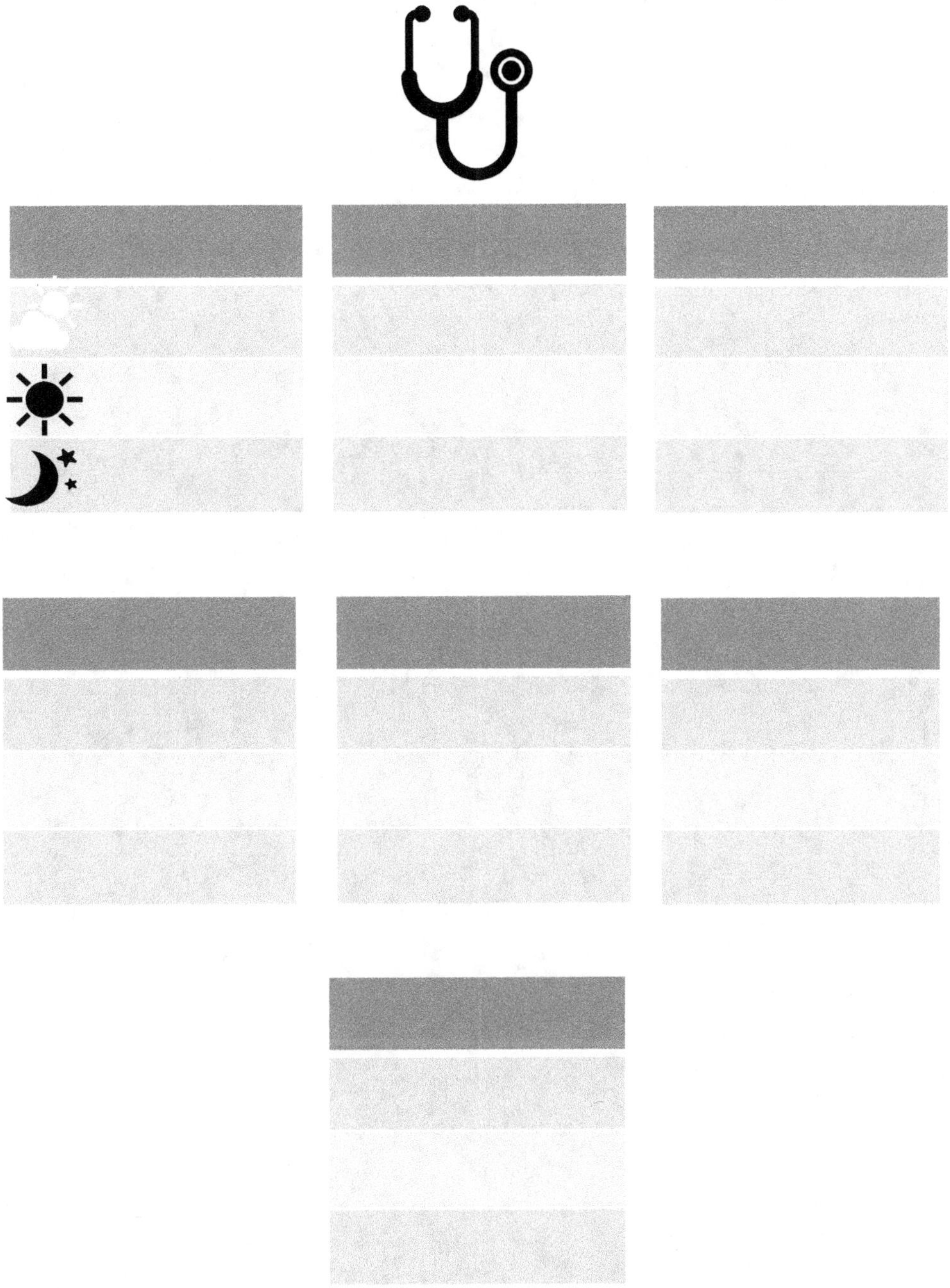

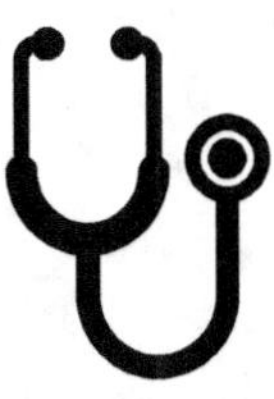

MEDICAL NOTES

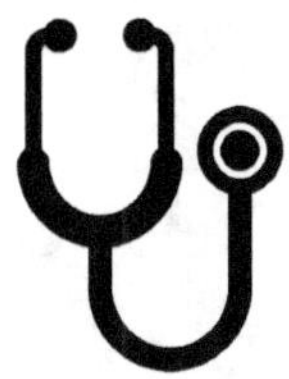

MEDICAL NOTES

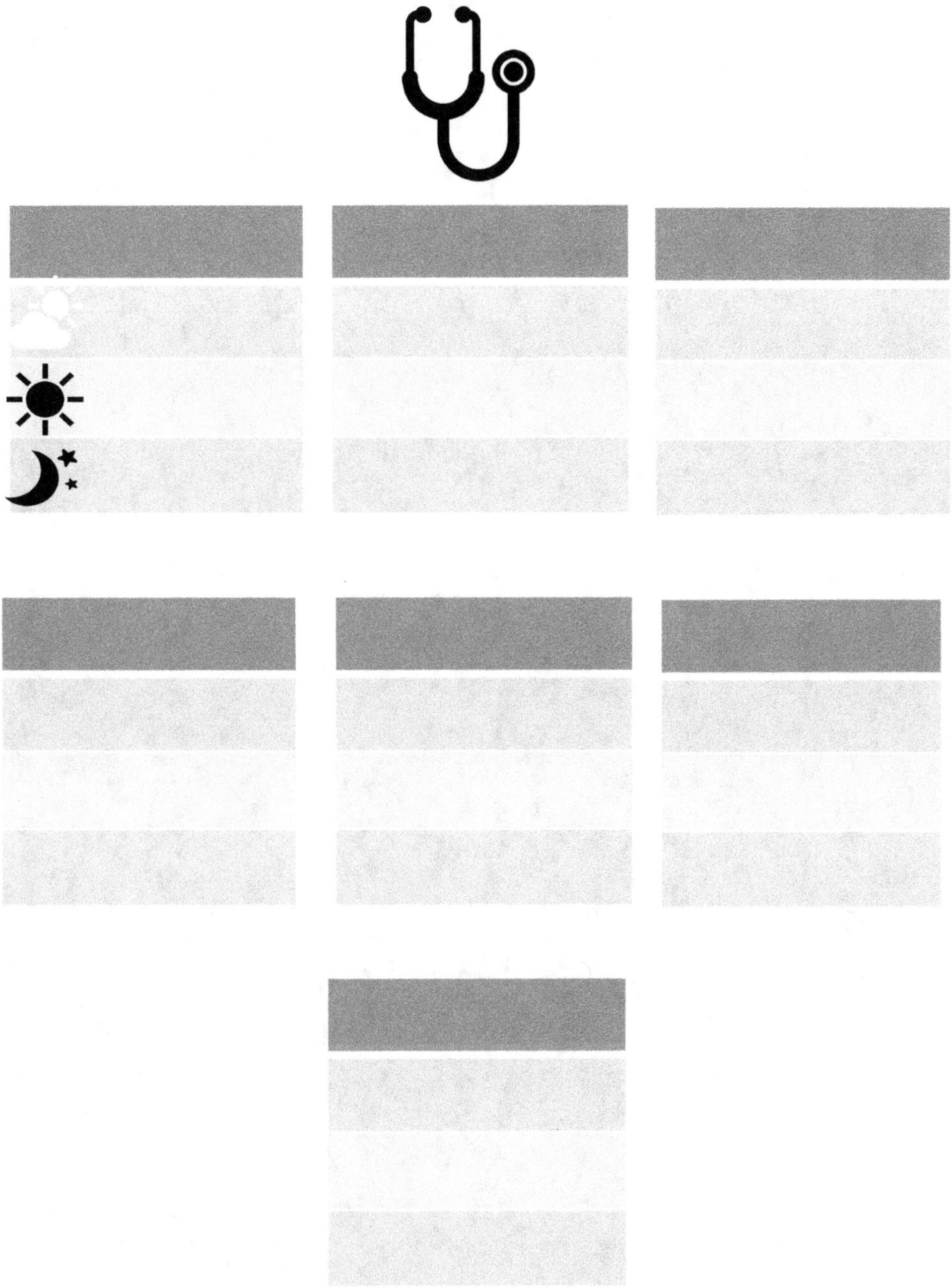

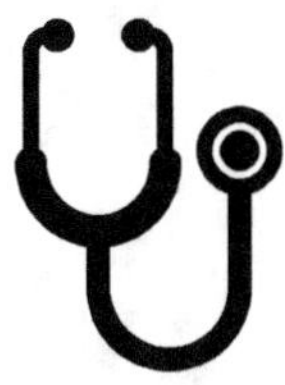

MEDICAL NOTES

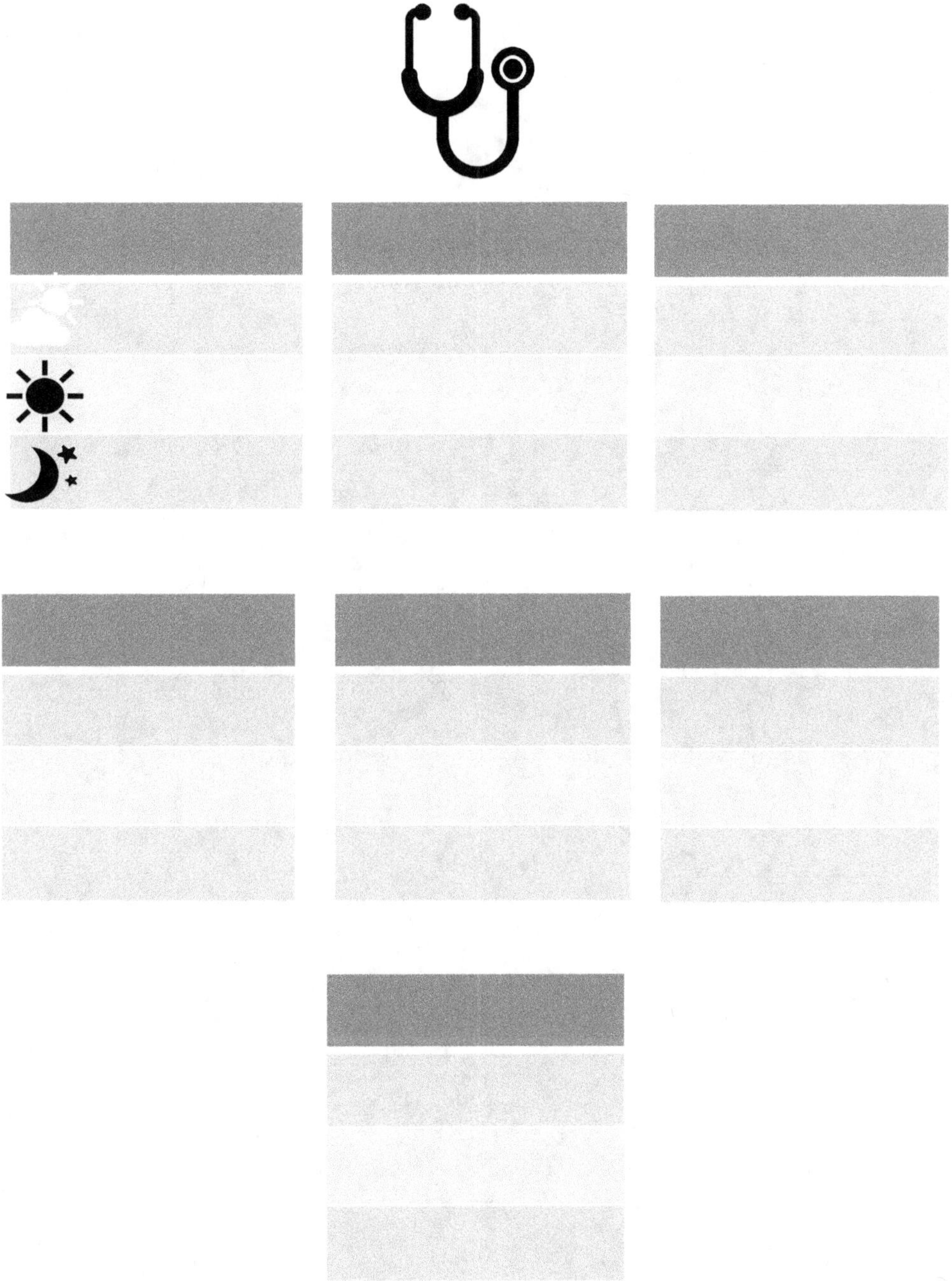

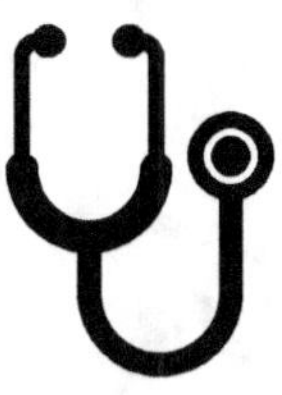

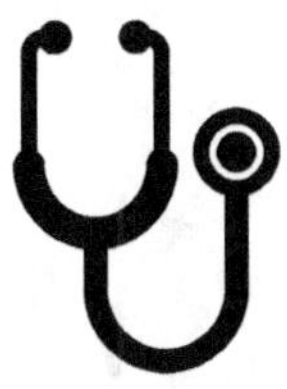

MEDICAL NOTES

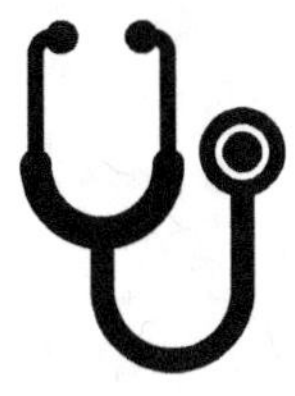

MEDICAL NOTES

MEDICAL NOTES

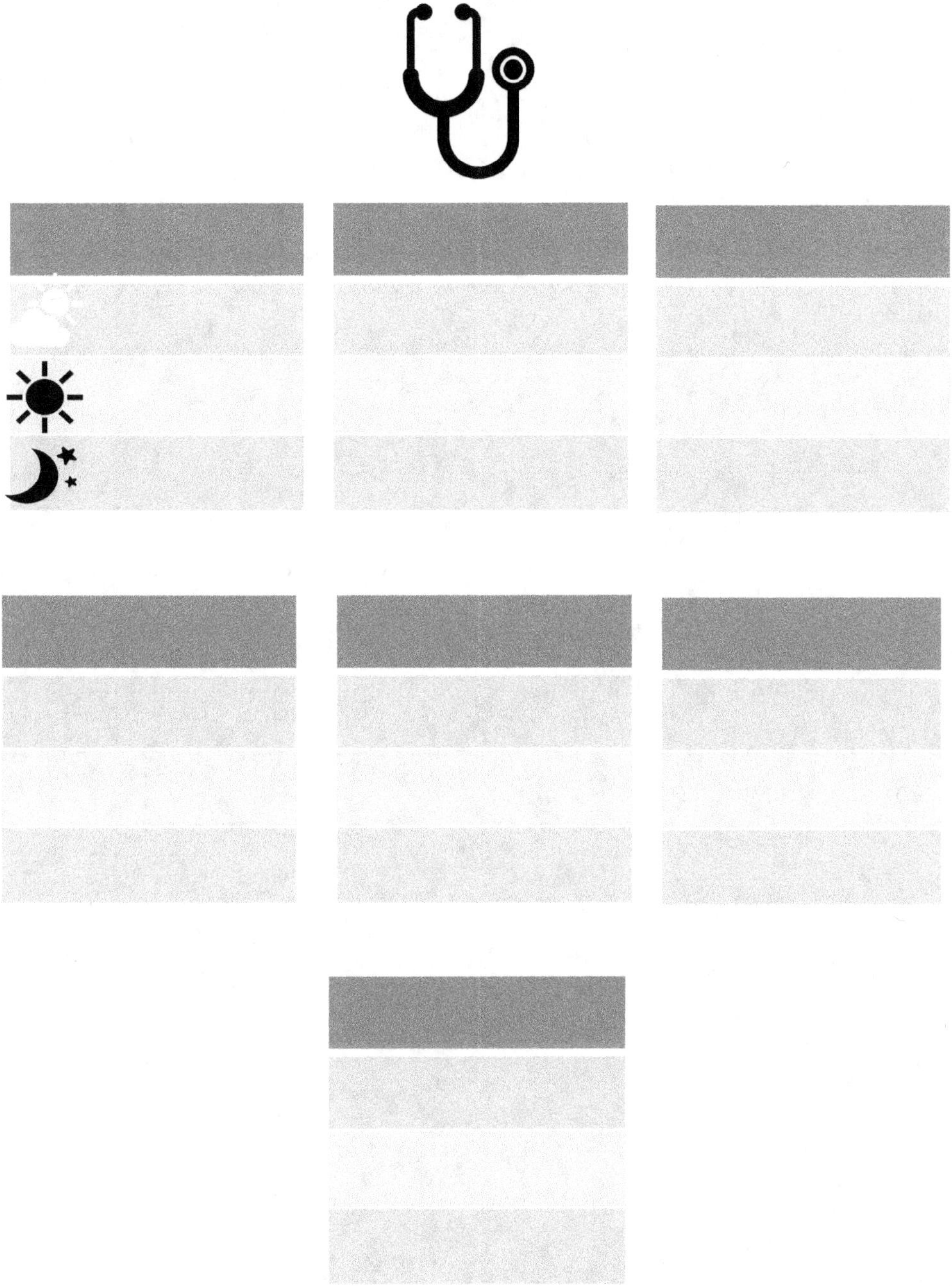

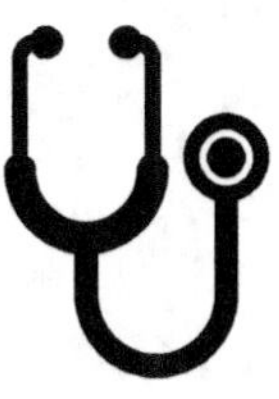

MEDICAL NOTES

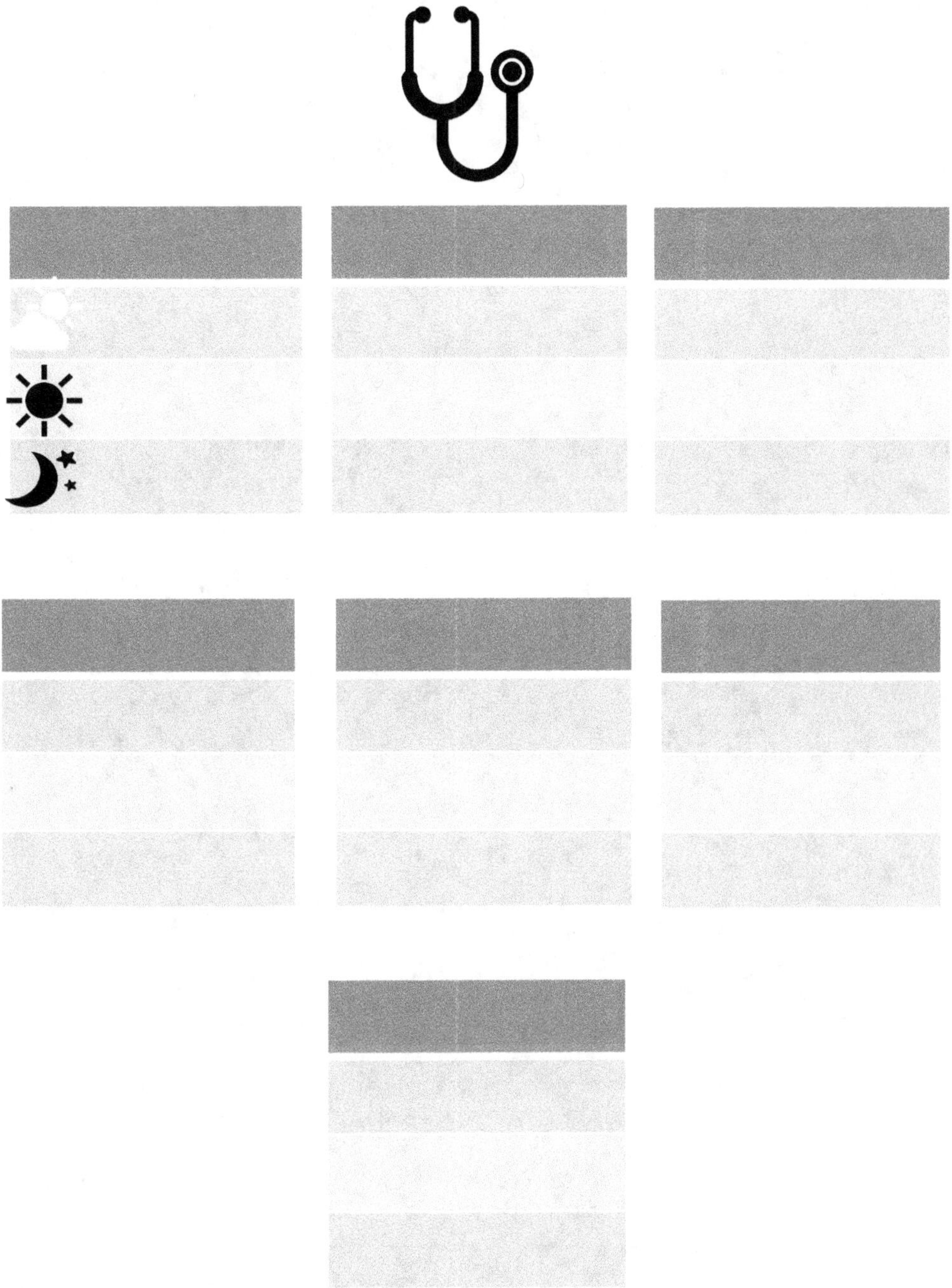

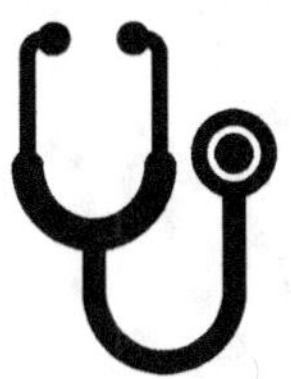

MEDICAL NOTES

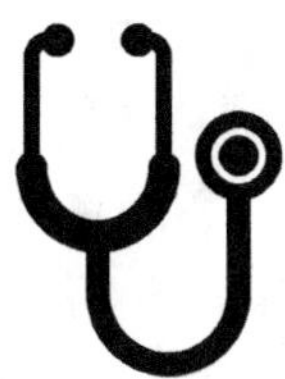

MEDICAL NOTES

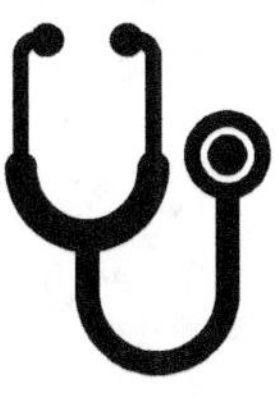

MEDICAL NOTES

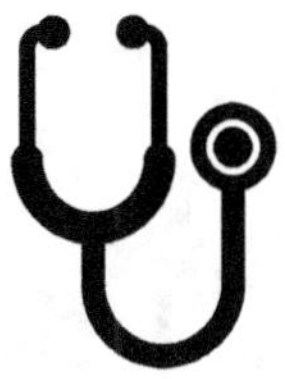

MEDICAL NOTES

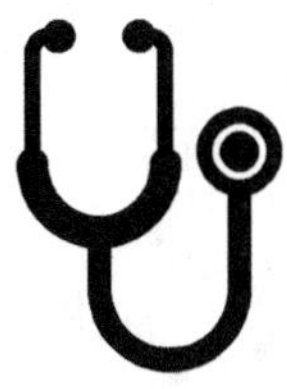

MEDICAL NOTES

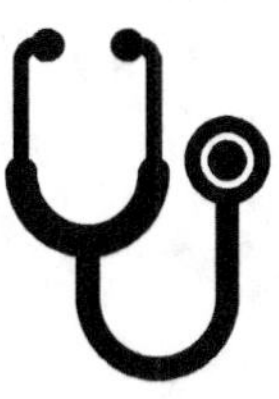

MEDICAL NOTES

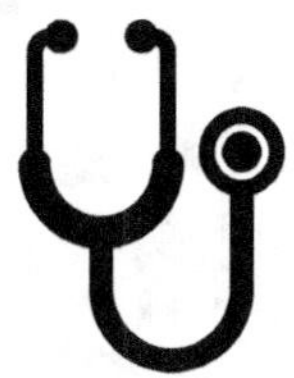

MEDICAL NOTES

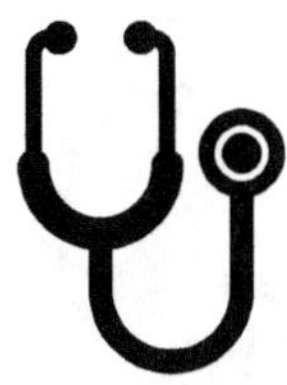

MEDICAL NOTES

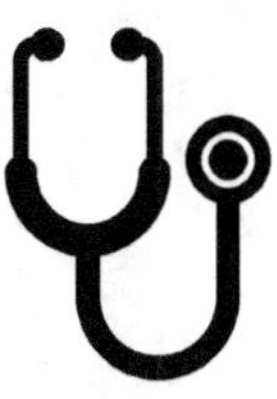

MEDICAL NOTES

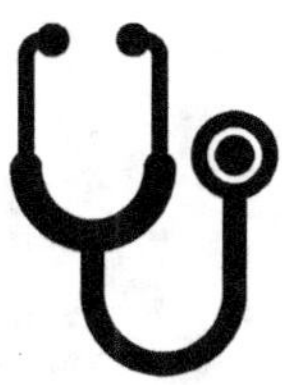

MEDICAL NOTES

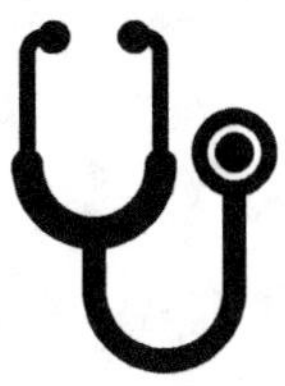

MEDICAL NOTES

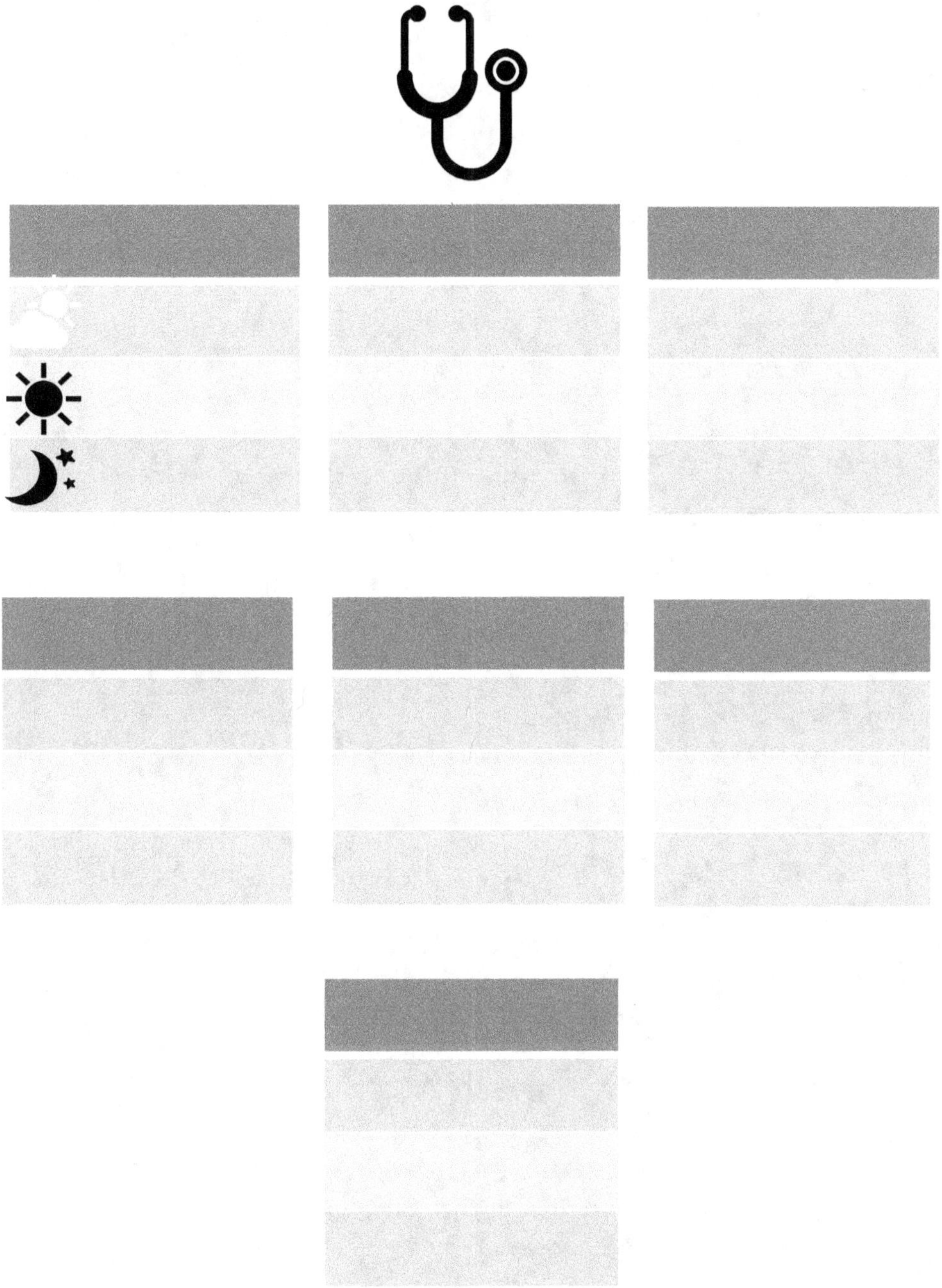

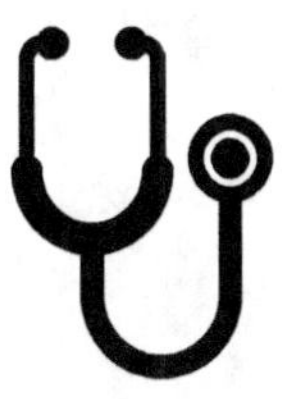

MEDICAL NOTES

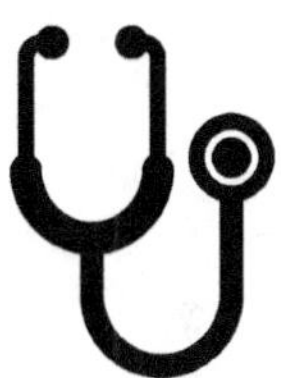

MEDICAL NOTES

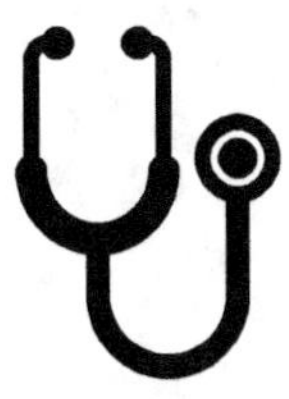

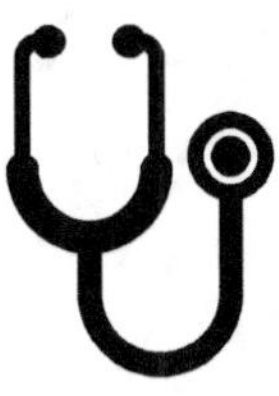

MEDICAL NOTES

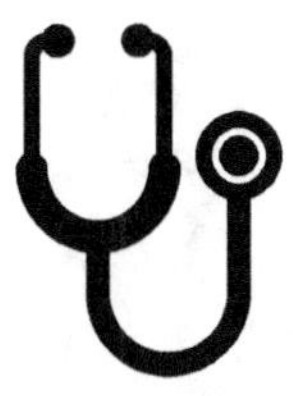

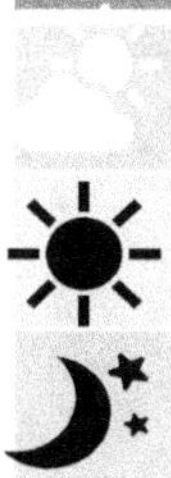

MEDICAL NOTES

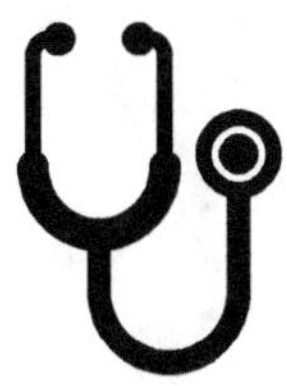

MEDICAL NOTES

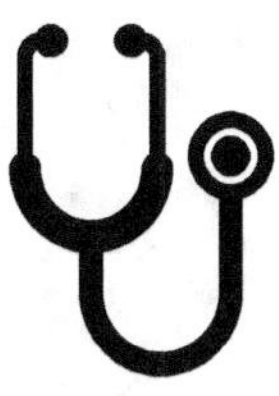

MEDICAL NOTES

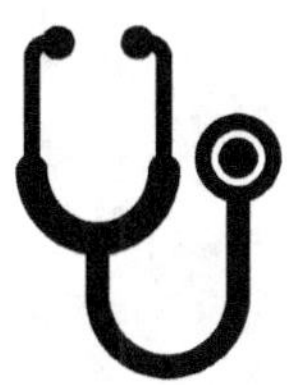

MEDICAL NOTES

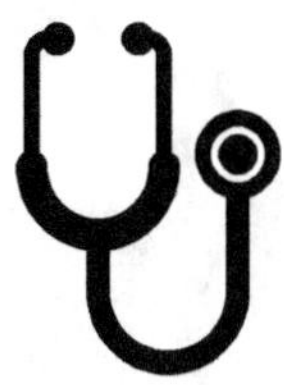

MEDICAL NOTES

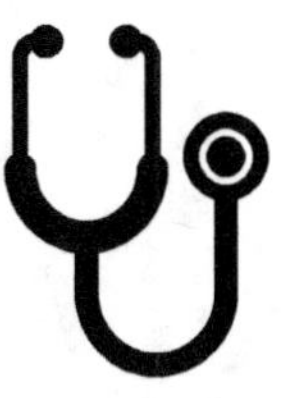

MEDICAL NOTES

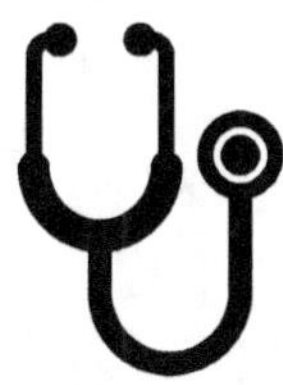

MEDICAL NOTES

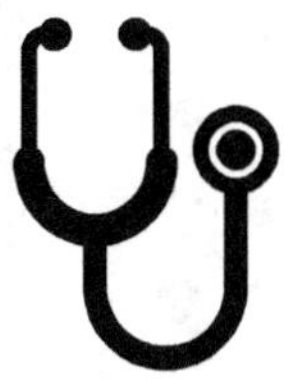

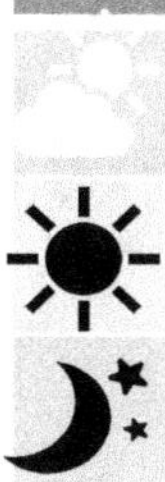

MEDICAL NOTES

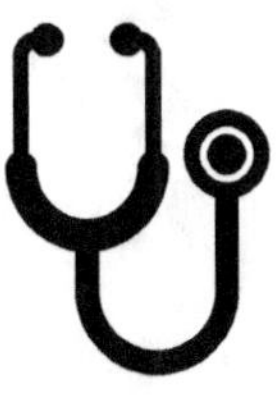

MEDICAL NOTES

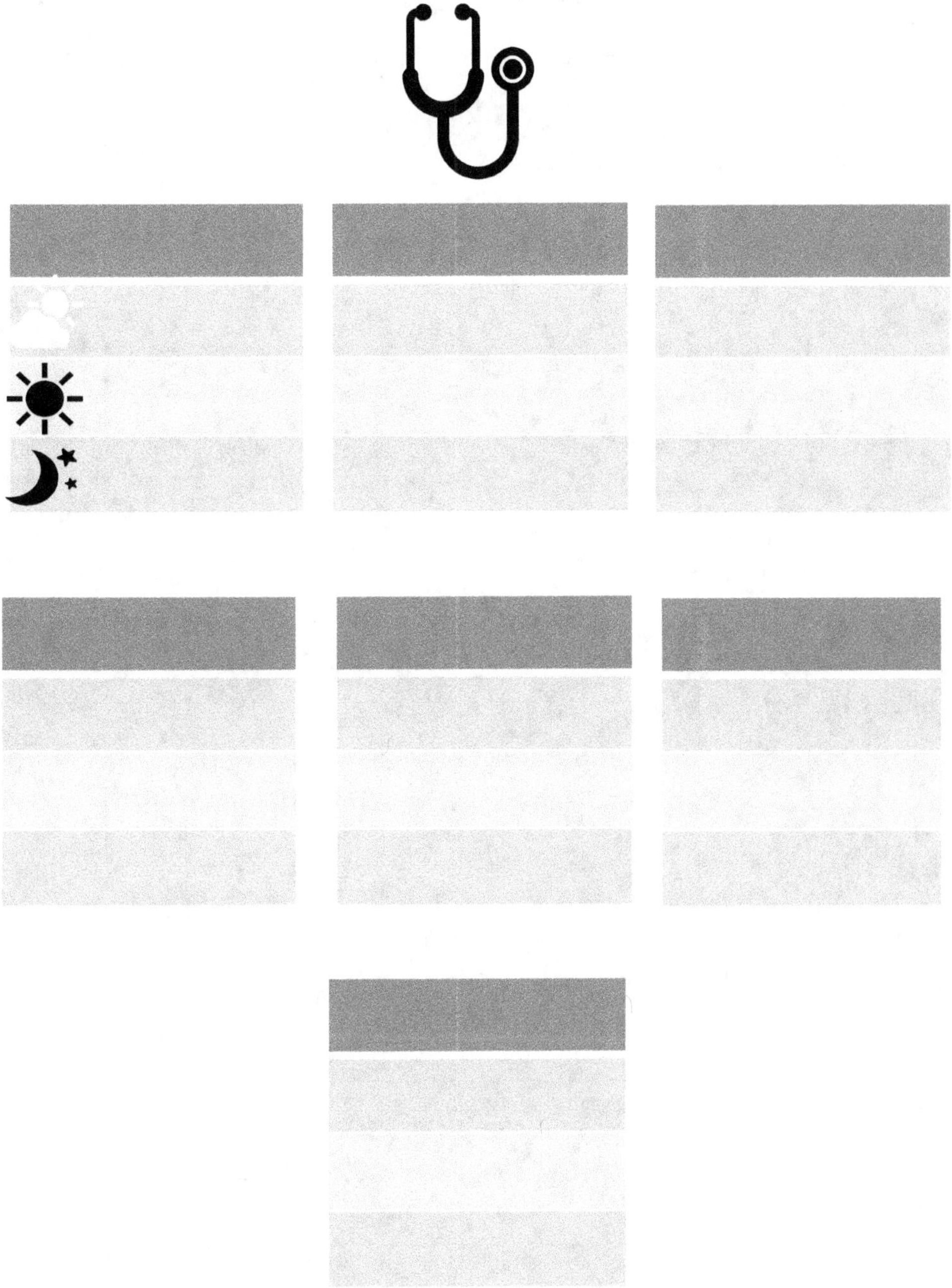

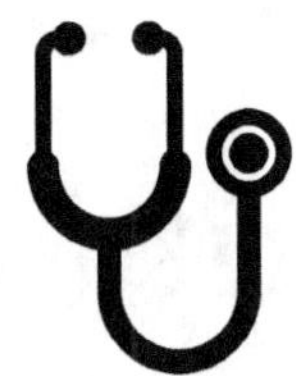

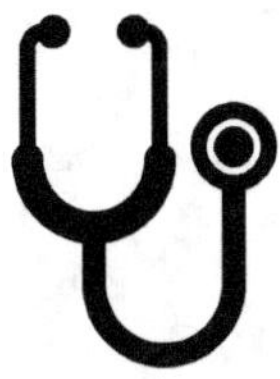

MEDICAL NOTES

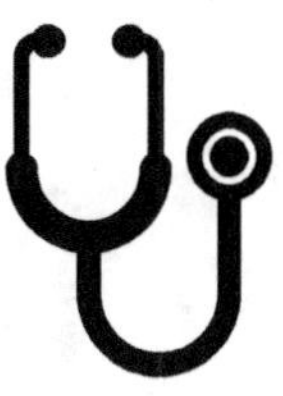

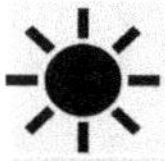

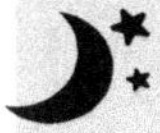

MEDICAL NOTES

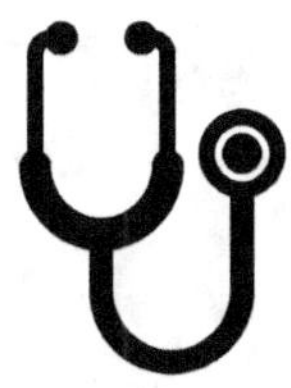

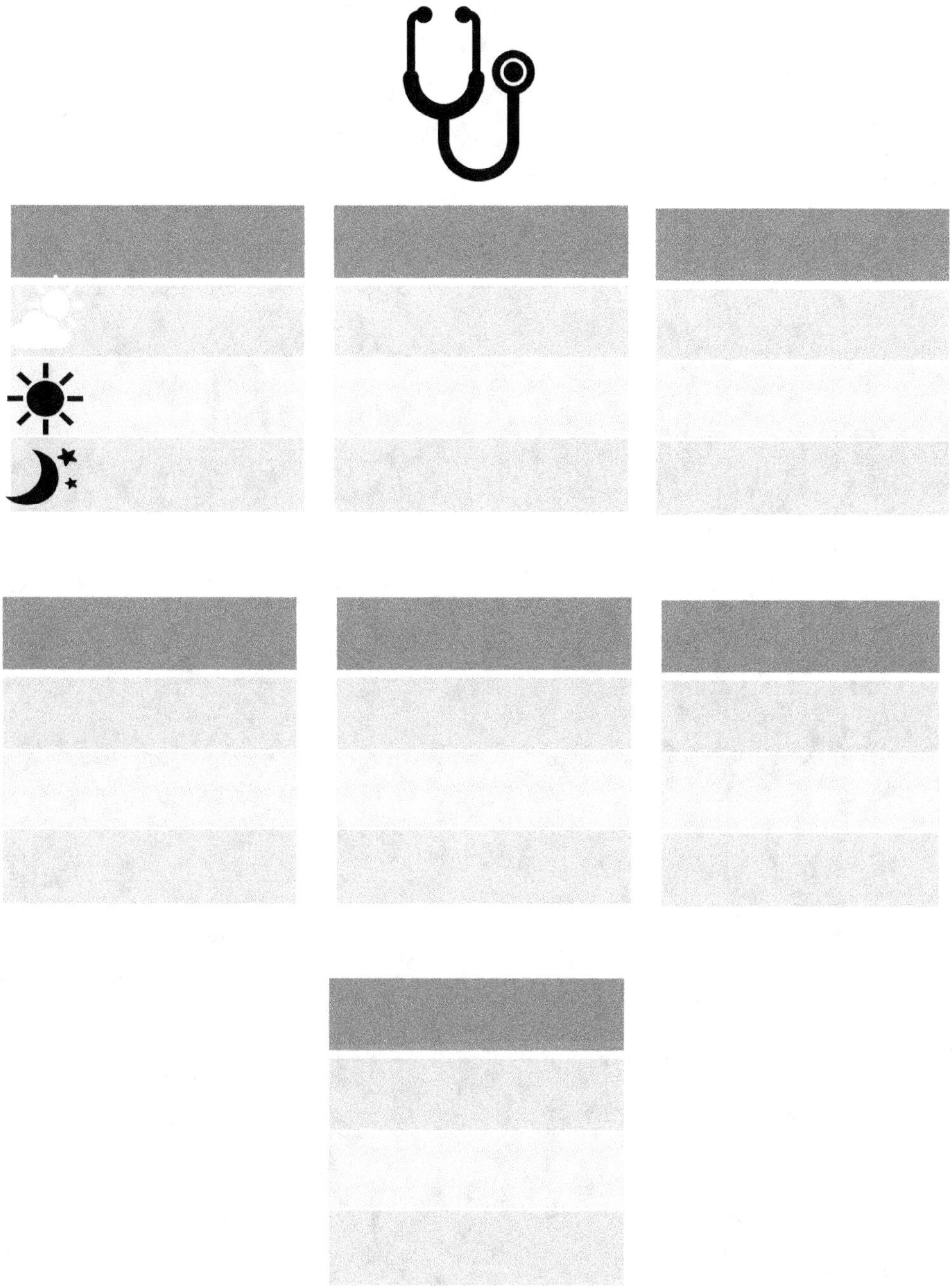

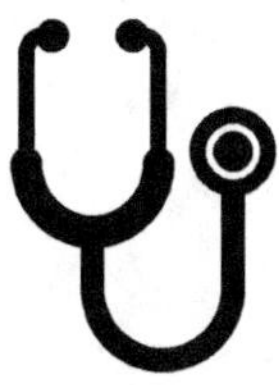

MEDICAL NOTES

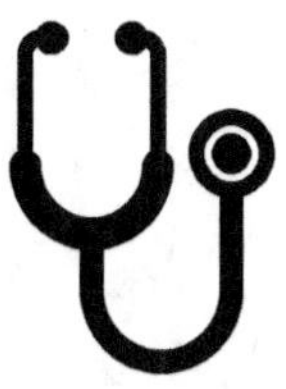

MEDICAL NOTES

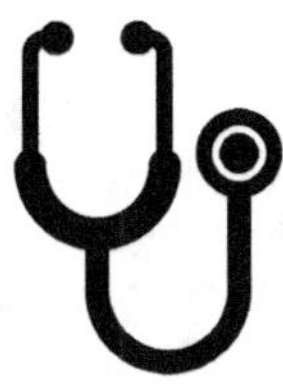

MEDICAL NOTES

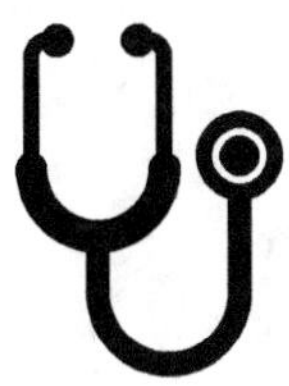

MEDICAL NOTES

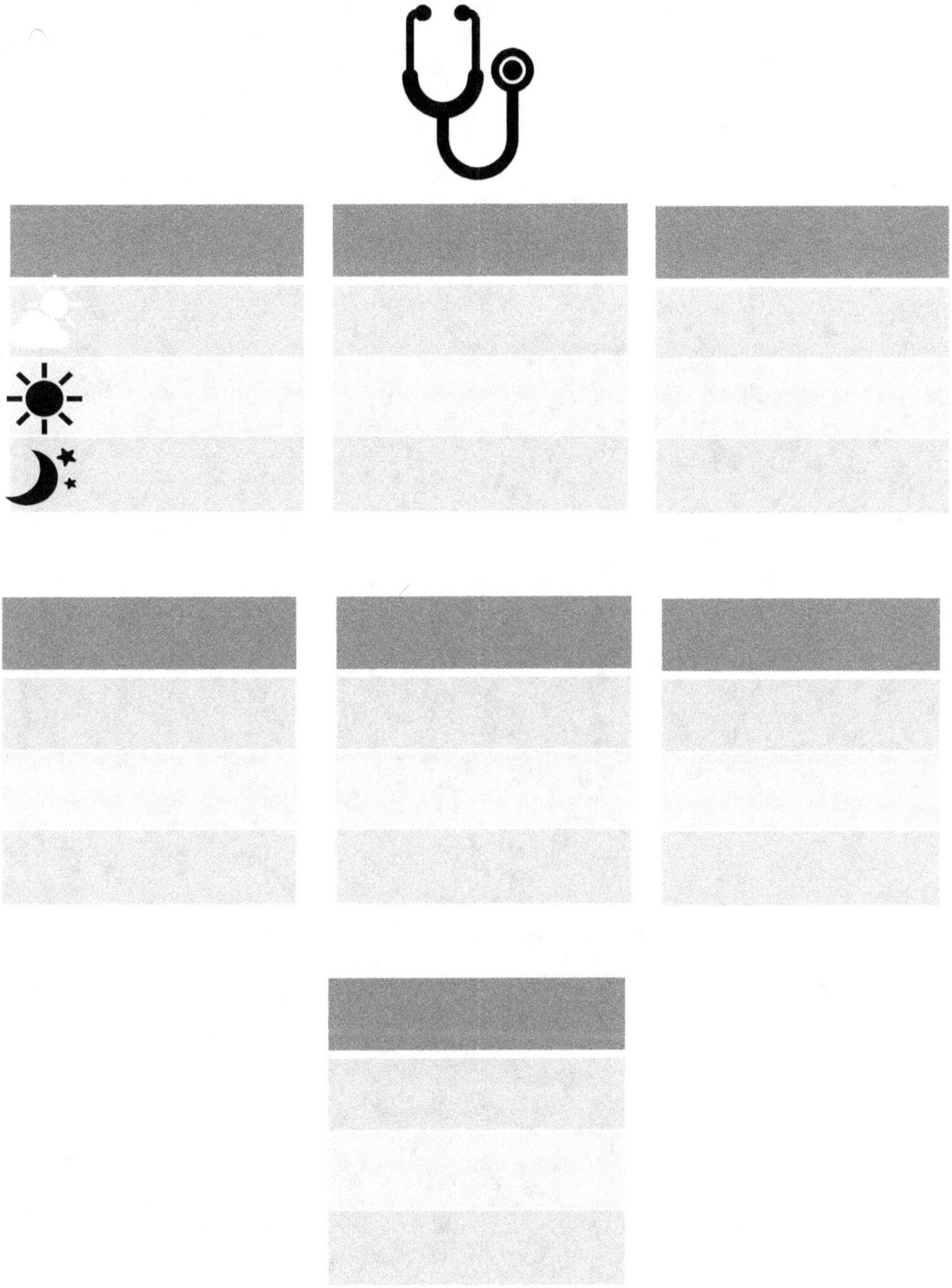

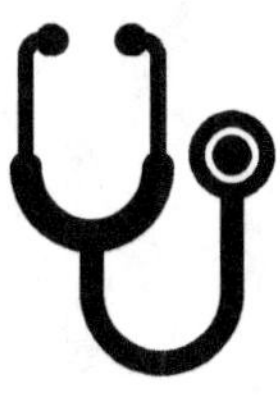

MEDICAL NOTES

www.ingramcontent.com/pod-product-compliance
Lightning Source LLC
Chambersburg PA
CBHW071229240726
48654CB00009B/972